Aspies Alone Together- A Survival Guide for Women Living with Asperger Syndrome

By Elaine M. Day

Table of Contents

About the Author 5
Introduction 8
What's Really So Different for Women on the Spectrum? ... 10
Diagnostic Criteria for Asperger's Syndrome 13
Part One- My Life 21
What Asperger's Is Like for Me 21
Childhood 24
High School Life 30
Adulthood 33
Part Two- Surviving And Thriving as a Female with Asperger Syndrome 42
Sensory Issues 43
Meltdowns 46
Social Issues 49
Dealing with Change 54
Relationships 56
Parenting 62
Employment 67
Depression and Anxiety 69
Bullying and Abuse 73

Getting the Right Help 76
The Gifts of Asperger Syndrome 78
Conclusion 79
Glossary of Terms 80
Acknowledgements 83

About the Author

While this section often comes at the end of a book or is found on the back cover, I find that it is relevant to the writing of this book for the reader to know who I am. At the time of this writing, I am a 33 year old Aspie who has only been diagnosed for a little over a year, though I have known for a bit longer.

My family history is a bit convoluted, and explaining it will help many parts of this book make sense. I was adopted shortly after I was born, but my adopted mom left and my adopted dad passed away when I was a year old, although I was already living with his parents when he passed. My grandma and grandpa were the parents I knew all my life, and they loved me unconditionally, even though a condition that, particularly because we knew nothing about it, made me incredibly difficult to deal with at times. My Grandma passed of kidney failure when I was 11, after years of sickness, and my Grandpa raised me until I was 16. The mom I talk about throughout this book is my biological mom, with whom I reconnected at the age of 20.

I grew up in much the same way as my peers. I was taught how to make friends and how to engage socially, and because of that that I was blessed with friends and the ability to fit in better than many males on the spectrum might without a diagnosis. I may have always stuck out like a sore thumb in some situations, but I had the social skills needed to survive, even if they didn't come naturally. Part of this is simply because I am a female, and part of it comes from growing up in the American South, where please, thank you, yes ma'am, and eye contact are drilled into your head the way a teacher might do with a specific math rule. My grandparents worked hard to instill me with manners and social skills, and I am eternally thankful for that.

With that said, life with undiagnosed AS was often hard. I often said or did the wrong thing (still do), and frequently I realized that I just didn't feel normal or much like my peers. I dabbled in the theory that I was an alien, wondered if being adopted meant that I just couldn't feel normal, or whether there was something inherently wrong with me. Like my AS hero John Elder Robison, there was even a time when I was desperately worried that the way I felt (and didn't feel) meant that I was a secret sociopath, destined to one day end up in prison.

Not fitting in didn't just mean not getting the cool table at lunch. It meant doing something against the rules in physical education one day and being treated to a large group of classmates singing "Blame It On Elaine" to the tune of a popular song at the time. It meant getting bullied my entire life. Told that my mom gave me away because I was stupid during ballet class, beaten up on the bus almost every day, and most importantly, the victim of sexual bullying at the hands of older kids and eventually adults. It's a dangerous side of being an Aspie, the increased likelihood of bullying and sexual abuse, and it is one that will be addressed in this book.

With that said, I feel that I have grown up into a functional and successful adult. I still need a therapist and psychiatrist to help me manage the symptoms of AS, but I am successful nonetheless. I have a strong, if small, circle of friends who understand me completely. I have a career that lets me be my own boss and that lets me take breaks when I need them, whether for an hour or six months. But most of all, I have a family. A beautiful wife (thank you Vermont for making that legal), two beautiful children, and a menagerie of pets who all constantly remind me that being wired differently isn't a deficit or a problem, but instead quite often a beautiful gift indeed.

Introduction

My ah-ha moment came in the middle of the night. I had gone to the bookstore and picked up a copy of a book called Look Me In The Eye by John Elder Robison. I had never heard of Asperger's, but the book looked funny, was on sale, and was written by the brother of one of my favorite authors of all-time. I started reading after my wife went to bed, and it wasn't long at all before I started finding myself in every word. Every page led to another ah-ha moment, another time I would elbow my dear wife and explain to her that I was practically reading a book about myself. Needless to say, she didn't get much sleep that night.

For many these days, there is no ah-ha moment so much as a diagnosis made at the suggestion of a teacher or day care provider or even a pediatrician. But for many adults with Asperger's Syndrome, we have been living undiagnosed for many years. This book is written for anyone and everyone, but primarily it is designed as a survival guide for women with AS who haven't had years of formal diagnosis, CBT, and help and for those of us getting diagnosed in our 20's, 30's, 40's, 50's, and beyond.

There are hundreds of books out there for people on the spectrum, but the vast majority of these books are aimed at males. It makes sense, as there are many males on the spectrum, but the large number of females on the autism spectrum means that we need resources, too. While AS is similar between the sexes, there are also many differences. For many females, we are taught social skills, or how to mimic them very early. This method of fitting in, even when it feels unnatural, can mask diagnostic criteria and can mean that many females go undiagnosed until well into adulthood when the deficits caused by AS start to cause problems. This can be in the workplace, in relationships, or elsewhere, but the simple fact is that for those who are wired differently, AS will eventually rear its head and it is critical that we see it for what it is and respond appropriately.

My goal with this book is multi-fold. In part, I want to tell my story and share with other readers how I have coped and how I grew up. I also want to create a sort of survival guide for others like me. And at the end of the day, I want to provide a good read for anyone who chooses to pick up this book and peruse its pages.

 It is my hope that it helps others find the strength and skills that I've had to form over the years with greater ease and that, if nothing else, it reminds all of you that you aren't alone. Even when isolation is the only thing you need in the world, there is a strong bond between us all and we are certainly Aspies alone together.

What's Really So Different for Women on the Spectrum?

It's hard to pinpoint all of the little things that make life as a female Aspie different. And part of that is in the cultural difference between the sexes. Little girls are more likely to be taught eye contact, pleases and thank yous, ways of engaging with adults and other children, and other social skills from a very early age. Social deficits are not something that cannot be overcome to some degree and that there is no diagnostic rule that Aspies can't make and be friends. With that said, however, a profound deficit in social skills and lacking peer relationships are criterion that are currently used to make a diagnosis.

So what happens when you have an entire gender of people for whom solo play is socially frowned upon? What happens when "boys will be boys" isn't an option and these lacking social skills are gained via rote memorization of responses, actions, and behaviors? For many females, it means missing a diagnosis of Asperger Syndrome.

Another diagnostic criterion used in determining if someone has AS is whether they respond with reciprocity in social situations. Again, many of today's young girls (and yesterday's, of course) are taught pleases, thank yous, and how to react to a gift or compliment (even if they don't like it) with gratitude or the appearance of it. Social reciprocity, eye contact, and even mannerisms are actually physically taught to us from an early age in an attempt to make sure that we develop into appropriately mannered young women, and the simple fact is that it can make diagnosing AS at a young age almost impossible given the current blanket criteria.

But with all this talk about masked criterion and what female Aspies are often NOT like, it is important to look at traits that are common among female Aspies. While these traits are not present in all females with AS, as we are all individual, they are certainly more common in females on the spectrum.

Female Aspies have a tendency towards hobbies such as reading fantasy novels rather than more male special interests such as memorizing train schedules. This adoration of fantasy also leads many children with AS to develop fantasy worlds. This is likely because we frequently feel the need to escape the world as it is, with its many stimuli and social pressures.

Also. while female Aspies certainly possess the ability to lie, we are typically honest to a fault. This honesty can lead to many problems. We can also be very naïve, which can lead not only to misunderstandings, but to being taken advantage of. With that said, we are also typically very deep thinkers, analyzing all of the things we see, do, and experience in great detail. While this can lead to anxiety, our ability to think logically and deeply about even simple things makes us excellent problem solvers.

Female Aspies are quite adept at putting on facades. We can mimic those around us, often with great success, in order to avoid seeming out of place. We mimic styles of dress, laugh when everyone else laughs (even if we don't get the joke), and copy what seems to be normal in the setting that we are in. This still creates a great deal of anxiety around whether we are getting it right, but this ability to camouflage can certainly help in social settings. It is important, however, to not allow our mimicry of others to enable us to lose touch with who we are as individuals, as self-acceptance is a critical part of dealing with and celebrating AS.

While there are certainly better and better tests being developed (and changes pending in the DSM), the diagnostic criteria certainly make it easier for males to be diagnosed and exclude many females who have been taught ways to cope with their own wiring differences. The criteria definitely work better for males, who are still the most commonly diagnosed but who may or may not truly make up the overwhelming majority of Aspies. There is no doubt that the science will catch up with the reality, just as we are now learning how many previously undiagnosed adults there are on the spectrum, but for many, having some resources in the meantime is critical.

Diagnostic Criteria for Asperger's Syndrome

Before we go much further, it is important to look at the formal diagnostic criteria for Asperger's Syndrome. This is the list that psychiatrists and other professionals currently use to diagnose AS, although these criterion often result in the exclusion of many females who warrant a diagnosis due to their ability to mimic social skills and special interests that are not as markedly different as many of those chosen by male Aspies.

[The following diagnostic criterion list is from Diagnostic and Statistical Manual of Mental Disorders: DSM IV]

(I) Qualitative impairment in social interaction, as manifested by at least two of the following:

(A) marked impairments in the use of multiple nonverbal behaviors such as eye-to-eye gaze, facial expression, body posture, and gestures to regulate social interaction
(B) failure to develop peer relationships appropriate to developmental level
(C) a lack of spontaneous seeking to share enjoyment, interest or achievements with other people, (e.g.. by a lack of showing, bringing, or pointing out objects of interest to other people)
(D) lack of social or emotional reciprocity

(II) Restricted repetitive & stereotyped patterns of behavior, interests and activities, as manifested by at least one of the following:

(A) encompassing preoccupation with one or more stereotyped and restricted patterns of interest that is abnormal either in intensity or focus
(B) apparently inflexible adherence to specific, nonfunctional routines or rituals
(C) stereotyped and repetitive motor mannerisms (e.g. hand or finger flapping or twisting, or complex whole-body movements)
(D) persistent preoccupation with parts of objects

(III) The disturbance causes clinically significant impairments in social, occupational, or other important areas of functioning.

(IV) There is no clinically significant general delay in language (E.G. single words used by age 2 years, communicative phrases used by age 3 years)

(V) There is no clinically significant delay in cognitive development or in the development of age-appropriate self help skills, adaptive behavior (other than in social interaction) and curiosity about the environment in childhood.

(VI) Criteria are not met for another specific Pervasive Developmental Disorder or Schizophrenia

Of course, as anyone with or who knows someone with AS can tell you, these criteria are not the whole of Asperger Syndrome. Here is a list of other common traits and features of AS, including many that are more common in females than males:

- 9 out of 10 people with AS have gastrointestinal problems (I've had surgery for mine)
- People with AS are typically more emotionally sensitive and immature than their NT counterparts
- People with AS tend to dress more for comfort than fashion and may not spend as much time on hygiene and personal grooming.
- People with AS may not have a strongly defined personality and may seem to change frequently to meet the needs of those around them.
- People with AS are prone to anxiety and depression.
- People with AS are often bullied or traumatized, increasing the risk for PTSD.
- People with AS often stim, or self-soothe, via rocking, foot tapping, or other repetitive motor behaviors. They may also do this when happy.
- People with AS are prone to anger or rage when they feel that they are misunderstood.

- People with AS often prefer the company of animals to people.
- People with AS tend to use control and routines to help manage stress and anxiety and will be very rigid with these rules, morals, and routines.
- Many people with AS are highly sensitive to medications that work well for NT individuals.
- People with AS are said to lack empathy, which would be better described as a deficit in the ability to show empathy.
- People with AS are often described as cold hearted because their words and intentions are often misunderstood.
- People with AS can experience not only meltdowns, but shutdowns in social situations, withdrawing entirely from the situation and becoming unable to continue the façade of social interaction.
- People with AS often struggle in traditional work environments and may have a hard time maintaining employment or even finishing their education.
- People with AS often have a high intellect and one or more very well developed talents or skills.

One area where AS has a profound impact on individuals is in sensory processing. For an NT, or neurotypical person, an itchy sweater or bothersome tag can be annoying. For someone with AS, it can be enough to trigger a severe emotional reaction. The same can be said for bright lights, busy social situations, loud noises, strong smells and tastes, and other intense sensory stimuli.

It is also worth noting that the definition of an intense stimuli is different for someone with AS than it would be for an average NT. For me, this is best described by my aversion to the texture of cotton balls and the squeal they make if you rub them. Most people can't even feel or hear it, but to me it is one of the most painful things on the planet. On what I call a "sensory day", I actually have to retreat to a special room in my house with blackout curtains, earplugs, a weighted blanket, and other sensory tools to help me cope with the sounds, sights, and smells that are a normal part of the day.

People with Asperger Syndrome tend to be very literal and have a hard time understanding sarcasm or inferring things that are not explicitly stated. I remember when I was little, I was eating chocolate covered peanuts and my Grandma expressed how much she wanted a peanut. Apparently she wanted a piece of candy, but I literally ate the candy off and gave her a peanut. I can still recall the sadness and disappointment she showed and how stupid I felt for not understanding what was really being asked of me.

Likewise, while I was very book smart at the time, I had a hard time understanding things that I didn't read or weren't told to me. We had a family friend who was dying of cancer, and she asked me for a kiss goodbye. In my mind, I knew if I did, I would get cancer and die, too, but I also wasn't supposed to turn down such a request, so I did it. I spent months waiting to die before I finally asked an adult how long it would take for me to catch the cancer.

Another feature of AS that is common is the meltdown. While many look at these as temper tantrums, they are actually reactions to being over stimulated in some way. I had a lot of meltdowns as a child. In fact, while they are getting better with age and therapy, I still have them as an adult.

A meltdown can trigger for almost any reason, but most have to do with the senses and the Aspie need for routine. A change in the plan for the day, being late to leave when a social event is supposed to end at a certain time, or a sudden sound like a fire alarm or even unplanned use of the vacuum can all trigger a meltdown in me. In fact, I used to have a journal left by my Grandma in which she stated that she would give anything to find out who made me so terrified of the vacuum cleaner. Oh, if only we had known.

Meltdowns can take a wide range of shapes and forms. It can be yelling, crying, head banging, hitting, or any other of a myriad of behaviors. Even for me as an adult, the shape of my meltdowns varies. Sometimes I bang my head until I am on the verge of a concussion, while other times I will cry, yell, or even throw an item that may have significant meaning to me outside of the meltdown. It's scary to me, and we work hard to manage my AS and my sensory input as well as to create schedules in order to prevent it from happening.

I've had meltdowns for as long as I can remember. As a kid, they got me into a lot of trouble, both at home and at school. Of course, when I was a kid, if I got spanked at school, I got spanked at home, and the school spanked me a lot. It's funny looking back, because I can remember every spanking I ever got, but for the life of me I can't remember the trigger that led me to yell, lash out, or otherwise implode.

Face blindness and difficulty recognizing tone of voice are also common problems for many with AS. Where most people can look at a face and understand what emotion is being conveyed, it simply doesn't work that way for many on the spectrum. The same is true for tone of voice. Sarcasm, anger, and other tone changes can often go unnoticed. Even as an adult, I can never tell when someone is being sarcastic or asking a question by making a statement with a lilt in their voice.

Aspies also have a tendency to get into trouble in school or even with the law. While we tend to have strong moral codes and convictions, we also live by our own sets of rules. For students, school troubles can arise for many reasons, including bullying from peers, rules that don't seem to make sense, the need to stim during class time, and even having a meltdown. Likewise, meltdowns, trouble with rules and authority, and other issues can lead to problems with employers and even the law later in life. As you will learn in this book, I was no stranger to trouble in school and once found myself in trouble with the law as well.

It's hard for girls with AS to grow up undiagnosed, even if I did eventually turn out to be a fairly functional adult. I was lucky enough to be a bit of a tomboy, which excused my preoccupation with baseball cards and my overwhelming urge to play baseball or play in the woods alone rather than socialize when given my options, but it was never easy. I was clumsy, aloof, couldn't say or do the right thing with my peers, and almost always the subject of ridicule by classmates even when I was the subject of adoration by teachers.

School was both tough and easy for me. I loved the work, the tests, and the learning, and my teachers loved that about me. But I also loved to do my own thing, to follow the rules that made sense to me, and often to go on ad nauseum about my interests while my teachers were talking- something they tended to loathe about me. My nickname from virtually every teacher I ever had was "The Mouth of the South", and I am positive that I never had a teacher, principal, or assistant principal whose paddle I didn't meet.

Part One- My Life

What Asperger's Is Like for Me

It's easy for someone to look at the diagnostic criteria and think that they have an understanding of AS, but the truth of the matter is that life with AS is completely different from normal life in many respects. While I will take a deeper look at various stages of my life in the next few chapters, I want to take some time to explain what Asperger Syndrome is like for me.

I guess the easiest place to start is to say that I have never felt normal. I still don't. Maybe that is because technically I am not- at least not neurotypical. I am wired differently from most. Most days, I relish this. It makes me very focused on what I set my mind on doing, gives me great strengths in my areas of interest, and in my opinion allows me to experience love, joy, and other emotions in a more intense way than others can, even if I cannot express them properly. When I get depressed or melt down in the middle of a social event, however, I admit I find it hard to see the blessings.

I do well with my friends and can socialize for small bits of time. I melt down from time to time, although less than usual and rarely in public these days. The grocery store and other crowded stores are definitely the hardest for me besides large social events. I am very intelligent and could read around the time I could walk, but cannot tell when someone is being sarcastic or making a snide remark. I don't read faces very well. I hate certain smells, tastes, and touches, including certain ways my wife can touch my arm. I am very hypersensitive and it bothers me to hear fluorescent lights or the sound of someone's pants rubbing together when they shake their leg. I hate the sound of pens clicking and the feel of cotton balls (just ask my mom, who was once hit in the face with a flying bottle of acetaminophen while driving because I touched the cotton).

I am good with computers, both building and repairing them. I love video games, sometimes to the point that I will shut out the world for hours or days at a time. I love to write, and have made a career as a freelance writer so that I can ghostwrite for others and not have to directly deal with people.

I try to be a good wife, but I have a lot of routines that make life harder for my wife, especially at bedtime. I hate change and have to know when events will end before I can be comfortable attending. I melt down if we are late to leave. I take my stresses with the world home, and it makes me melt down over little things, and sometimes my wife gets caught in the crossfire, thinking I am melting down over something she has said or done. Really, though, I melt down at home because it is the one place I feel safe and secure.

I try to be a good parent, but often miss family meals because of the sound of everyone chewing. I sometimes miss the importance of concerts and other big events because they seem trivial to me when I have things to do. I am rigid in my rules, and sometimes I think it makes me more of a disciplinarian (grounding and time-outs) than I should be.

I try to be a good person, but I melt down as soon as someone isn't listening to what I am trying to say or I feel misunderstood or belittled. I have a hard time with rules that make no sense to me. I struggle with situations where logic tells me to do one thing, but it is expected of me to do another.

I have a sensory room where I eat my meals and spend a lot of time. I sleep in this room when I am overwhelmed and find it to be a place of solace in a world that makes absolutely no sense to me a lot of the time. I keep weighted blankets, eye masks, and other items in here to help me retreat from my senses as well as the world.

Despite all of these things, as well as the many that I have forgotten, however, I am a lot like everyone else. I feel happy and sad. I get angry and I feel elated. I am sad for the misfortune of others, even if I can only feel empathy by imagining that it is happening to me. Asperger's makes me different in a lot of ways, but in most ways, I am just like everyone else.

Childhood

Before explaining my childhood from an Asperger's standpoint, I want to just spend a little time explaining my childhood overall. It was, of course, the most formative time in my life, and in many ways it was one of the best.

I was raised by my grandparents. We did lots of things together, and they were in every way my parents. Grandpa taught me how to ride a bike, Grandma and I used to play Atari and Commodore 64 together, and they taught me the lessons and skills I would need my entire life.

I lived in the same house my entire childhood, and Grandpa still lives there. I think it helped give me a sense of roots and is why I really long to find the place where I will spend the rest of my own life.

Grandma and Grandpa were always doing things with me when I wasn't playing alone in the yard or with a friend. We took walks, swam in the pool, and generally did everything together. It was wonderful, and there was never a moment that I didn't feel loved and even spoiled. I even had my own go-kart track in the field beside our house.

My life started changing around the fourth grade, as my grandma's kidneys started to fail, but I was shielded from a lot of it at first. She was on dialysis three days a week, but when I went, they would either let me sit with her and watch the little portable TV so that it didn't seem scary, or grandpa would take me to the park next door. One of the few times I stayed in the lobby, an older gentleman had a heart attack and I had to bang on the nurse's window for help. It was scary, because I had just been talking to him, but I was able to act logically in the face of a crisis. I can still remember the names of all of the regular patients at the center, from the gentleman in question to the lady who always traded Harlequin romance novels with my Grandma.

When I was in fifth grade, my Grandma had to go to a hospital in Dayton, Ohio for treatment. I had no idea how sick she was, and was concerned that she would miss my play. I stayed with friends of the family while she was gone, and their two sons and I had a good time, so I guess I really wasn't worried that things could go wrong. When they finally came to get me, I remember very clearly my Grandma telling me that I almost didn't have a Grandma after something went wrong at the hospital. It was the scariest thing I had ever heard, yet still she put on the façade that she was fine.

Her last Christmas was in 1990, and it is one of the worst memories of my life. Somehow, in the hustle and bustle of the holiday, she had managed to buy us all the world, yet nobody had a gift for her. I can still see the look on her face. Shortly after Christmas, in January, she had to leave to go to a hospital again. This time, I stayed with my nursery school teacher and her family. I remember talking to Grandma on the phone whenever she was able to call and check on me, but eventually she went into a coma as her system started shutting down. On January 26, I woke up for church and my nursery school teacher was standing there with a strange look on her face. She told me that my Grandma had died overnight. I was in shock and had no idea what to do or feel, so I went with them to church as usual.

I don't remember a lot before the funeral. The house was packed with family members who talked in hushed tones and said things they thought I couldn't understand. The one memory I do have is of my oldest cousin taking me outside and singing a song to me about how hard it is to say goodbye. It was the most comfort I felt since everything happened, and it probably the last time that, for even a second, the hole left behind by my Grandma wasn't there. I still feel it to this day.

The summer after Grandma died was spent with a family member in another state. I remember that summer well, but it wasn't a good one. I was made to sleep in the basement near the dryer, where it would keep me awake, and I didn't sleep very well. My accent made me the object of ridicule, and my main purpose seemed to be to clean and to cry on command. I was told that Grandpa thought I didn't cry enough after Grandma died and that if I didn't cry more, he was going to lock me away in a hospital. I know as an adult that this wasn't true, but at the time it really scared me. I tend to be very honest and blunt, and I took my family member at her word. It wasn't until the day I called him and explained everything that was going on, including being slapped by an adult for slapping a child that was harassing me that he found out how bad it was going. He came and got me in record time.

Shortly after Grandma died, Grandpa also started publicly dating a new woman. Today I love her more than I possess words for, but at the time, I hated her. I remember being so mean to her. I would say and do awful things, and I just wanted her to get out of our lives. She tried very hard to get me to come around, and eventually just to tolerate me, but I never relented or made it easy until I was an adult. To this day, I apologize every time I am there to visit and thank the heavens that she has been able to forgive and even love me.

Around this time is also when our new neighbors moved into the house that Grandpa originally built for my great grandmother. One of the neighbors was a gay man, and he took me under his wing and took me in like his own child. I adored him, and we went everywhere together. We saw all the latest movies, watched the coolest television shows, and basically cultivated my obsession with all things pop culture. We are still friends, and we spent much time together well into my teenage years.

Middle school was where life really started changing. All of my friends started moving into different cliques, and I didn't fit into any of them. Sixth grade was also when I started dating my first girlfriend, and I remember one student cornering me in the locker room to tell me that all of the gays should be put in a boat, sailed into the ocean, and blown up. I had friends, however, and they were good ones. In fact, the best friends I remember from middle school are still my friends today and that is something I am very thankful for.

Looking at the criteria in the last chapter, it is easy for me to explain how Asperger's affected my childhood. Despite being enrolled in ballet, theater, karate, gymnastics, beauty pageants and many other activities by my Grandma, I was never quite the social butterfly I was intended to be. I had friends, but I preferred to spend my time talking to adults. By the age of three, I was already reading on my own and learning to write, and by the age of five, I was tutoring children nearly twice my age in reading. My scores were off the charts for the tests they had at the time and I was enrolled in gifted programs where, once again, I preferred the company of my teachers to that of my peers.

Today I know that the verbal abilities and the way I spoke were a part of Asperger's commonly known as "Little Professor Syndrome", but as a kid I guess I just thought adults had more to add to a conversation and were less interested in play and other interactions that made little sense to me.

As far as special interests, I have always had one. For a while, it was collecting GI Joe action figures and letting them kill one another for hours on end, then it was my chemistry set, then an electronics kit that let me build all sorts of gadgets- but eventually I discovered baseball cards- a passion that held me in its grip for nearly a decade. I would organize and reorganize my cards by team, by batting average, by player position, you name it. I brought them to school, where they were the only thing I wanted to talk about, and I even had my own booth at the local flea market starting when I was around ten so that I could sell my cards. Today that interest has grown up (though I still collect), and my focus is primarily on restoring old furniture and World of Warcraft, but I can't think of a time in my life where there hasn't been a single focus that took up all of my conversations and attention.

High School Life

By the time I got to high school, I was a mess. Pressure to be social was at an all time high, and my failures in this area had never been more evident. Friends were few and far between, and the majority of my friends were grown men who were either gay or who had been coercing me into sex since I was in early middle school. It's ugly, but it's life.

I did have friends in high school, and it is important to make a note of that. I was always the weird kid, but I did have friends. In fact, the few friends I had were great to me. They knew I was weird, but they were the kind of people who just didn't care. It's one of the blessings of AS for me. The friends I made then, the ones who would defend my awkward behaviors, often at the risk of their own skin, are still my friends today, and I am blessed for that.

I also found ways to, if not fit in, to keep the number of people who actively hated me to a minimum. One thing I learned by watching my peers my entire life was that everyone liked someone who could make them laugh. I took that to heart, because I wanted nothing more than to be the kid that everyone liked (or wasn't afraid of), so I became a smartass. I was pretty good at it, too, much to the dismay of my teachers. I can't count the times that I was told that it made no sense that such a smart girl could be so bad. But I got laughs and smiles from my classmates, and for me, it was worth the trip to the office every time.

By high school, bullying had reached a peak. I was getting my tail kicked on the bus every day just for being me and because I wouldn't tell due to the fact that many of my tormentors would threaten my family or threaten to kill me if I did. As an Aspie, I tend to be pretty naïve, so I believed them. I was getting my tail kicked at school for looking at people the wrong way (I didn't know any better, I was just looking into the classroom). It was a nightmare. I was getting my work done and making great grades on the work I did, but my preoccupation with my first girlfriend meant that I wasn't doing homework, which didn't make sense to me since I already knew the material.

It's funny. I could make A's in any class I even made a halfhearted attempt to study in, but when it came to geometry, even all the help my teacher could give me wasn't enough to wrap my Aspie brain around the concepts. I was blessed that she passed me with a D, and although to this day she probably thinks I didn't want to learn geometry, the truth of the matter is that I still can't make it make sense.

Skipping class became the norm for me in high school. I knew the course material and I didn't feel like listening to all the snide remarks made at my expense, so it made sense to me to stop going. I would show up on test days, but if I could leave without getting caught, you can bet that I wouldUp until now, I probably hold the record for most days spent in in-school suspension (which I also skipped), and my Grandpa had to come and convince the principal not to throw me out more times than I can count.

During this time, my meltdowns evolved into cutting sprees. I would take whatever I could find lying around and cut my skin over and over and over, only to realize after the meltdown ended how badly I was hurting myself. This was also around the time that I started experiencing depression and making several attempts to end my own life.

I made it through to my senior year of high school and was on track to graduate. Then one day I was walking through the math building and looked into my math teacher's classroom. Two girls decided that I was looking at them funny and jumped me. Thanks to my school record as a juvenile delinquent (all of which was for skipping school or talking in class), I was deemed to be the instigator and threatened with being sent to a school for kids with behavior problems (the school where they sent kids who brought weapons to school or otherwise committed serious and dangerous violations), and that was my last day of high school. I dropped out and never looked back.

Adulthood

It's important to note that during the last year of my doomed foray into high school, I experienced some life altering events. My first girlfriend had been unfaithful and had gotten pregnant, so I gave up pretty much everything to help take care of her and the baby. As a bright girl with a promising future, this didn't sit well at home and I ended up running away to live with them in a trailer and thus began my early adulthood. Looking back it was stupid, but I'm not sure I could morally make a different decision even knowing how it all played out.

Asperger's has always had a huge impact on my relationships. With no understanding of the fact that I even had sensory issues, I was in a constant state of overwhelm. This was especially true when my girlfriend and I were spending every waking moment together taking care of a child and trying to make a life. It was volatile and at times even violent. We were both too young and too vulnerable to be adults yet, especially when I had no idea that I was wired differently, and ultimately the relationship was one that I am certain scarred us both for life, though I will always wish her the best.

My relationships, up until and including my marriage, have always been volatile. It wasn't until shortly after meeting my wife that I learned about AS, so I have always been prone to meltdowns and outbursts when overstimulated, and when you are in a relationship that involves being together a great part of the time, getting overstimulated is anything but uncommon.

Shortly before I turned 18, my Grandpa let me cash in the bonds and CDs left by my dad when he died (in my infancy). I bought a house and a car (81 Vette because I was practical) and worked hard to do the right thing. Unfortunately, I was also 17 and had no idea how to be responsible. Within a couple of months I had blown all of my money on friends that appeared (and disappeared) out of nowhere, taken out a mortgage, and put myself in a position where I had no way of paying my own bills. By now, my girlfriend was living with someone else, although we still shared visitation of her son, and I was living a nightmare.

When I turned 18, I received a box of paperwork that included my Grandma's journals, letters to my dad asking why he never came to visit me, citations he got from the military for misconduct, and a copy of the record of the accident that killed him. I read that paperwork every day, letting it shape my self-esteem and letting it mar the image of a man I had martyred in my mind since I was small. In October of 1999, I lit that box on fire in the middle of my living room and walked away. It was a singular moment born of depression and emotional overwhelm that changed my life forever.

After lighting the box on fire, I went to my first girlfriend's parents' house, where I slept on their couch. When the police came to the door to tell me that my entire house was on fire, I had no idea that they had told my Grandpa that I had probably burned to death inside. In fact, I only recently learned this. What I did know was that there were dozens of vehicles and people, all asking me questions, and all clearly looking to make me into a villain. From here, it spiraled out of control pretty quickly, and when they asked me if I did it to collect on the insurance it sounded a lot better than telling them that I had snapped over a few pieces of paper so I said yes. Little did I know that this meant that I would be charged with both arson and insurance fraud. Nineteen years old, and I was a felon. My life was getting better every day.

During the month I spent in jail, I once again got beaten up every day. Then one day they brought in a woman who had been arrested for murdering a senior citizen. She told me the story of how it happened and the microphones picked it up. This meant that I could be asked to testify against her, which her lawyer wasted no time in telling her. She made it clear that she was going to get the death penalty and had nothing to lose, so killing me would be fun. I had never been so afraid in my life. I decided to kill myself before she could.

The people at the jail apparently have rules for people who attempt suicide, so I spent a couple of days in a room with no windows or doors all by myself. The guards would make the door click very loudly every time I got to sleep in order to keep me up, and I could hear them laughing. These are the same police that once said after they were called to an intense argument with my girlfriend in which they tackled me into the street and smashed my face into the pavement, "hey, if you can't arrest a real man, let's arrest a fake one".

Luckily for me, my suicidal ideations meant that the jail had to transfer me to a mental health facility for supervision. It's called the Baker Act in Florida and it means that they can hold you for up to 72 hours. I stayed for a year.

It would be great to say that this is where I was diagnosed with Asperger's Syndrome. It wasn't. For that, I still had another 13 years to wait. In fact, the hospital in Florida was a nightmare. But it was better than being murdered in a jail cell. And it was the first time I realized that something might be wrong with me, something that could be fixed. It was also the first place where nobody treated me like I was bad or a miscreant or a delinquent.

During my stay in the hospital, they tried on diagnoses like shoes. Depression, anxiety, bipolar, psychosis, you name it. I must have tried 50 different meds, only to have each one fail spectacularly. I know now that meds affect people with AS differently than many others, at least in many cases, but at the time, I just thought that whatever was wrong, meds certainly weren't the answer.

I had lots of meltdowns in the hospital, but they were always chalked up to side effects or to whatever was wrong with me. I was once again getting bullied, albeit this time by patients. My AS symptoms were out of control, and somehow nobody ever picked up on it as a possibility. The only thing that made me feel better was spending time with an Alzheimer's patient who remarkably came to remember my name and my room, and I spent every waking moment with him... even when he had to be put in the locked ward due to his violent outbursts. For some reason he would never hurt me. We kept in touch for over a year after I was discharged and he was moved to the state hospital.

An amazing thing happened to me while I was in the hospital, and it changed the entire course of my life. One day, I answered the ward phone and a strange accent came over the line. "Is Elaine there?", the caller asked. I stated that I was indeed Elaine and I heard the four words I had always dreamed of but never envisioned hearing, "This is your motha (she's from Boston, R's aren't her strong suit)". We talked for about an hour. I learned that I had a younger brother, two grandparents, numerous aunts, uncles, and cousins, and a mom who loved me and wanted to meet me. We talked frequently and wrote letters during the rest of my stay, and when I was released I was put onto a Greyhound bus to meet my mom for the very first time.

The bus ride itself was interesting, for sure. At one point, our driver pulled over on the side of the road and quit his job, leaving us stranded there. At another, a transsexual person had put her feet on the seat of the man in front of her. The man complained and the passenger said "Do I look like a man to you?" The response was "No, but you sure sound like one", and a brawl ensued. At another point, an older gentleman who had been on most of my two day journey noticed that I hadn't eaten, so he got on the bus from one of our stops and handed me a box of chicken and potato wedges. It was so moving and thoughtful that, despite being a vegetarian at the time, I ate it with gusto and a renewed faith in humanity.

The best part of the two day bus ride, however, came at the end. Before finally falling asleep for the first time in three days, I happened to tell the woman beside me that when we got to Albany, I would see my mom for the first time. I woke up, excited, as we arrived in Albany, and it took me no time to recognize what looked like my own eyes and facial structure. When I ran up to hug my mom for the first time, I heard a massive roar of applause behind me. Apparently, my seat companion had told the entire bus what was about to happen and they had all gathered in anticipation of witnessing one of the biggest moments of my life. And it made it all the greater.

I ended up moving in with Mom and my brother, as well as her landlady, the landlady's two kids, two dogs, and a cat. Three of us shared a room. It was hectic, and Mom and I often had moments. We didn't fight, I was simply unable to tell her intent from her face or tone of voice, so I always took that northern bluntness as a sign of anger or frustration and reacted in all the wrong ways. I still have that problem, especially up north where sentences aren't punctuated with things like sugar, darlin', please, or other words that indicate the mood behind them. I don't understand faces and tones of voice, and it often leads to problems, even with my wife.

Meeting Mom and moving to Vermont gave me many opportunities. For starters, people are more open minded here, both to my quirkiness and in a deeper sense. I grew up in an anti-gay, often racist town, and moving to such a progressive state really made a big difference in my self-esteem and how I felt about humanity. More importantly, however, the move gave me a chance to change who I was and the direction my life was heading in.

My adult life has had many milestones. I spent many years writing poetry and a few months getting paid to read it aloud at places like Mount Holyoke and Yale, only to learn that my fear of public speaking meant that I was going to cry and have trouble making words every single time. I have had a number of relationships, all hallmarked by meltdowns, overwhelm, and eventual breakups over the volatility that comes with never taking a sensory break or learning that I cannot deal well with change and strong stimuli. But the biggest milestone in my life was one I never planned for, and it has led to life altering moments and discoveries I could never have imagined.

A number of months after a breakup, my friends convinced me that I really needed to start dating again. I got an email from a woman who seemed great. Two kids, a love for the same foods and activities as me, and a great personality. We started talking back and forth and it turned out that we had attended rival high schools back in Florida. In fact, we had crossed paths numerous times without ever meeting. We decided to go out for sushi. We've been together ever since.

It took only two months for Gayle and I to decide to get married. Everyone we knew told us what a terrible plan it was, and some so-called friends even went as far as to advise me to separate our finances and get away while I could. Thankfully, I didn't listen. Gayle, Monkey Boy, and The Girl (I am using the monikers I bestowed upon my children because I am uncomfortable giving their names in a publicly available book) are my entire world, and I don't think I could ever be the person I am without them.

I moved in with Gayle about a month after we met. It took no time at all to become a family, although there was a time when The Girl was worried that I was taking Gayle away and had fits every time we were together. Yet every night, she would beg me not to leave.

When I met Gayle, I had spent the past few months working insane hours and making more money than I had ever seen in my life. I had just come off of disability at the end of a previous relationship and started writing as a freelancer, and success was coming in ways I had never imagined. It was a huge shock to the system when, after moving in with a wife and two kids, I was no longer able to maintain that level of work. I kept writing, but at a much slower pace. Eventually, my wife left her career to come home and help me start and grow a writing business and help me get back on track, but until we learned about AS and did something about it, that simply wasn't the answer.

That's where the ah-ha moment mentioned in the beginning of this book comes in. The night I read "Look Me In the Eye" changed everything. Not instantly, of course, but it started a chain of events that is still making me better every day.

Once I read that book, I begged Gayle to read it. We started learning everything we could about AS, and the more we learned and the more we looked at other family members and their traits, the more it seemed like AS just might be the source of my differences. I started asking questions of Grandpa and my old friends, and everything just fit. I had long had a Facebook friend telling me that he thought I was on the spectrum, but until I read that book, I thought that he was crazy.

Since learning about AS, my wife and I have done a great deal of research. She has hand-made me a weighted blanket in Star Trek fabric, I have started medication to handle meltdowns and anxiety, and I have undergone CBT and other therapies as well as a brief hospital stay. By teaching my kids about AS, they have become more understanding and can even recognize when I am oversensitive or overstimulated before I do and can give me warning and space. Learning about Asperger's Syndrome has changed my life, and in the remainder of this book, I want to use my experiences to help change yours.

Part Two- Surviving And Thriving as a Female with Asperger Syndrome

In this section of the book, I want to take a look at some of the different aspects of AS as they pertain to females. I also want to look at some of the tips and coping tools I have used and still use, as well as issues that commonly affect people with AS. Here, we will look at sensory issues, meltdowns, bullying and abuse, relationships, dealing with change, seeking help, and more.

I hope that this section of this book will provide those of you with AS or who know someone with AS with a box of coping skills that you can use as well as a greater understanding of the challenges that those of us with AS face. The simple fact is that we live in a neurotypical world, and our wiring simply makes it harder for us to do many things that come naturally to others. With that said, it is important to realize that AS can also give us many gifts that many neurotypical individuals simply are not capable of.

Sensory Issues

One of the hallmarks of Asperger Syndrome is that it involves a disruption in the processing of sensory stimuli. We get overwhelmed easily, whether it is via sight, smell, taste, touch, sounds, crowds, or simply being in a busy and stimulating environment. In this section, I want to look at some of the coping strategies and tools that I use to help me deal with overstimulation.

One of the biggest recommendations I have for women with AS is to create a sensory toolkit that you can carry in a purse or other bag. This can include any number of things that help you cope. For example, my sensory toolkit includes sunglasses, ear plugs, a smooth stone I can rub my hands over to keep from rocking or making other repeated gestures, chewing gum, and a stress ball that my daughter made from a balloon filled with sand that I can squeeze when I am on the verge of melting down.

I also have both a weighted blanket and a compression vest. Deep pressure is an incredibly effective tool for calming the senses, and both my blanket and my vest are very important parts of my life. My blanket can be used any time I am overstimulated or near a meltdown, while my vest allows me to go into public and socially overwhelming situations with a much greater sense of calm and self control. They can be quite expensive, but both the vests and the blankets can be made at home if you (or your spouse) happen to be handy with a sewing machine.

Dealing with sensory issues is made much easier by my sensory kit and tools, but this does not make the problem go away. There are still days where the sound of the kids running and screaming through the house or the smell of a spice-heavy dinner will overwhelm me. During these times, I have to rely on deep breathing, speaking up for my needs, and anxiety medications to help ensure that I can cope with these issues.

One thing that I have been blessed with and that I recommend for any Aspie who has access to an unused space is to create a sensory room or space. For me, it is my office. I maintain black curtains and a wide range of sensory tools in order to allow myself a retreat when I am overwhelmed. I also have a sign for my door so that others know when I am in need of sensory time. For those without an extra room or office, a sensory space can easily be made in a bedroom, garage, shed, or other quiet space, especially if you make family members aware of your needs.

Because this book is primarily aimed at female readers, there is one point that I feel is relevant to share. For me, and I suspect many other Aspies, the hormonal changes that come along with menses bring about an increase in sensory overload and meltdowns. Sometimes, simply being aware of this can help you prepare yourself and your loved ones for the pending need for greater quiet time, isolation, or sensory time and space.

Sensory issues can be incredibly hard for women with Asperger Syndrome, but they can also be effectively dealt with. Taking the time to make a sensory kit and put it in a purse or other convenient location can make a big difference. Make sure that you are doing what it takes to meet your needs and work hard to create a sensory free space to help you in times of overwhelm.

Meltdowns

Meltdowns are a big part of life for some women with Asperger Syndrome, and they can be huge. For some women, myself included at times, overload can come in the form of a shutdown, or a total retreat from people, sensory stimuli, and the world at large. Other times, however, it can be like a full force hurricane during which all you can do is wait for it to pass.

It is important to note that a meltdown is not a temper tantrum. Instead, it is a physiological response to outside stimuli. This can be a change in routine, too much sensory input, a disagreement that has gone too far, or a myriad of other triggers. What neurotypical people who care for someone with AS need to understand, however, is that once a meltdown starts, it is already past the point of no return. Yelling, talking, or trying to actively stop the meltdown will only cause it to escalate and it is best to let it safely play itself out.

For me, a meltdown can come in many forms. As I mentioned before, I may bang my head, retreat (shutdown), or yell. Sometimes I throw or break things when a meltdown isn't recognized and the stimuli continue. I don't intentionally harm people or animals, but many of my favorite possessions have been lost in the blind rage of a meltdown. I have broken cell phones, monitors, and even prized family possessions (my own) in the midst of a meltdown, only to still cry at the thought of it months later.

When it comes to meltdowns, some of the responsibility lies on those closest to us. While we are ultimately responsible for our own behavior, it is important for those around us to realize when a meltdown is occurring and to do what is possible to stop an argument, remove sensory stimuli, and simply be understanding of what is going on. I can tell you from personal experience that a meltdown can happen anywhere, from a family reunion or parade to the grocery store or the living room. I can also tell you that no matter how embarrassed it may make our loved ones feel, the shame of a public meltdown is almost always worse for the person with AS. When I melt down at the grocery store, it is all I can do afterward not to abandon the cart and never return to the store. I hate the awkward stares, and the looks at my wife wondering why in the world she would be with someone who would lose it when the store is out of a particular kind of macaroni and cheese. At least, that is what I feel like they are thinking.

During a meltdown, I am not thinking. I may say and do things, but I am not in control of my actions or behaviors. That is why it is so important for the meltdown to be allowed to stop.

It is important for others to realize that some time needs to pass after a meltdown before it or the triggering event can be discussed, lest it start all over again. For meltdowns that began over an argument or similar trigger, Aspies will also often need to be reminded or told to apologize, especially when we feel that we were right in the argument. Furthermore, after a significant meltdown, most Aspies will need at least a day to fully recover. Meltdowns create a fight or flight reaction and create a great deal of stress and chaos, and it can take the body and the mind some time to process and deal with this.

Some research shows that women are more prone to crying and temper meltdowns than their male counterparts, even in public, including throwing things, yelling, or even banging their head. I know this is true for me. Learning how to manage the triggers that come before a meltdown and planning for outings in advance can go a long way in helping to prevent these and in lessening their severity.

Social Issues

A big problem for most Aspies comes in social situations. There is a common saying that the easiest way to cure an Aspie is to put them in a room by themselves. I have to say that this one is definitely true for me. I have never had a meltdown while home alone, unless I was on the phone during a stressful phone call.

One area where female Aspies frequently experience social problems is in making and keeping friends. While we are often much more adept at developing social skills than male Aspies, eventually people are able to see that our social skills are more of an act of memorization than something that comes naturally. Awkward conversations, inappropriate comments, and a lack of ability to read faces and detect sarcasm can lead to self-consciousness and can have a social impact on many females with Asperger Syndrome.

Social problems can also occur on a much larger scale when it comes to social events. Many Aspies long for friendships and social interactions, only to find themselves under tremendous stress and anxiety when placed in a social gathering or event. For me, gatherings such as family reunions where there will be strangers or parties where I know I will be expected to maintain conversations with people I do not know well causes me significant anxiety. Even meeting a new doctor or attending group therapy can be incredibly overwhelming for me. When possible, I learn as much as I can about people who will be attending so that I can have points of conversation ready if need be.

With friends, I have found that I have been lucky enough to be surrounded by people who are willing to learn about Asperger's, as well as those who just naturally embrace my quirks. This isn't always the case, however, and sometimes it is necessary to educate someone or even to terminate a friendship if it turns out that your symptoms become the object of ridicule or if your friend refuses to accept your needs for routine, planning, and the need to leave an overwhelming situation. For many females, the ability to naturally observe and intellectualize appropriate social behaviors makes it easier to obtain friendships, although maintenance can still be quite difficult.

In friendships, I have been quite lucky. My best friend Shannon can actually tell when I am overwhelmed or nearing a meltdown long before I can. She is also great in social settings because of this ability. She often lets me know when I am arguing a stupid point with my wife due to my constant feeling that being right is more important than being happy and works with me to teach me when there is more value in shutting up than in continuing a debate or argument. According to her, I think like a man, but in truth, I just think like an Aspie.

While I met Shannon as an adult, I have always had good friends at my side. My best friend growing up, Kim, was unfailing in her ability to put up with me. I can't count the times she had to defend me for saying or doing the wrong thing in the wrong group or situation, yet without fail, she always did. My surrogate brother, Josh, has also been one of the truest friends the universe could ever provide. Friends like these are real blessings for me, and I am not sure what I would do without them. My circle of friends is small in number, but each of them are close and I can't imagine my life without a single one of them, even when we go months without talking at times.

In terms of social events, I find that planning is an absolute must. When my family goes to an event, or when my wife and I go to a party, a restaurant, the theatre, or even to a store, we make a plan. We plan what we need to buy, what we expect the event to be like, how many people will be there (for things like family gatherings), and most importantly, what time we will both arrive and leave. This gives me the feeling of control I need and gives me a set time when I know that the event will be over. My wife has been incredibly good in this respect, making sure that we leave events on schedule, even when I know there are times that she wishes to keep socializing. I work hard to accommodate this desire, but in events where I am socially overwhelmed, it is often impossible. Five o'clock means five o'clock, and by 5:02, I am usually in the middle of a panic attack.

It can often be harder for females to experience social gatherings simply because it is easier for us to give the appearance of fitting in. We are incredibly adept at smiling and holding conversation for as long as we are able, but we are also prone to crying and having major meltdowns when we are no longer able to hold up the façade or become overwhelmed.

Advice

To help overcome these sorts of social issues, there are a few things that you can do. For starters, it is important to surround yourself with supportive, caring, and understanding people. The right friends can make a big difference, and they can provide a great deal of security and comfort in social situations.

Another great tip for surviving social situations and gatherings is simply to observe people when you can before speaking. I have a seemingly natural ability to blend into a crowd and go unnoticed when I need to, and this allows me to watch people and hear their conversations before I have to talk to them. In doing this, I am better able to understand their interests as well as their sense of humor or mannerisms.

Last, I always recommend making a plan before any social gathering. Write it down and keep it in your pocket if you need to. My notes often include not only what time I expect to leave, but what the event will entail as well as positive affirmations about my ability to get through the event and even to enjoy myself while I am there. In CBT, they call these Coping Cards and they can be incredibly effective tools.

Building a social wellness toolbox is something that can benefit all Aspies, especially female Aspies. Our quirks are often far less tolerated due to the way females are expected to act in public, and having a strategy can help ensure that you better fit in. We may often feel like square pegs trying to fit into round holes, but with a bit of planning you can bend the event to fit your needs rather than trying to fit in where you feel that you don't belong.

Dealing with Change

Change is a big hurdle for most Aspies. This can be a change in circumstance, the loss of a pet or loved one, a change in routine, or a change in plans. In some cases, even the smallest change can be enough to cause a meltdown. For most Aspies, the need to control our own worlds stems from being in a world that is so far beyond our control and often our understanding. What is easy for others is difficult and draining for us because we live in a world we don't always understand and that we have to work hard to fit into.

There are many strategies to help us deal with change. While some changes take much time to adapt to, learning to deal with smaller changes can be easier. One helpful tool comes from CBT and involves testing your thoughts around the change. Ask yourself some basic questions such as what will really happen as a result of the change? Is this result something you will survive? What advice would you offer a loved one experiencing the change? The truth is that we have a habit of catastrophizing what will happen when things and routines change.

With that said, I also know that this is easier said than done. To this day, I can still meltdown at the drop of a hat when a planned event runs late or my bedtime routine is interrupted or delayed. Even positive events, like an unexpected visit from a good friend can throw my life into chaos. This can easily cause me to become tense or even agitated. In fact, there are times when my reactions can be described as ballistic. I need order in my life, and many other women on the spectrum are just the same.

Sometimes we know that a change is coming, whether it is a move, a change in our jobs, a change in our relationships, or simply an upcoming event. In times when change is both coming and inevitable, catastrophizing and worrying can be of little benefit. Instead, it can be very helpful to envision life after the change and to gather as much information as possible on what things will be like after the change occurs. This could mean asking about new job duties, researching the area around a new house or apartment and taking photos so that you can decide in advance where everything will go, or planning the times you will arrive at and leave an event and what you will talk about or do while there.

Relationships

While there are many female Aspies who choose to remain single and/or celibate, many of us choose to enter into relationships throughout our lives. For many of us, it is only when we are with a long-term or live-in partner that the symptoms of AS start to finally become more problematic. This is one of the reasons that many high functioning female Aspies aren't diagnosed until adulthood.

While I am in a same-sex marriage, I realize that most women enter into relationships with the opposite sex. To ensure that I do not exclude anyone in my writing, I will choose to use the term partner rather than boy/girlfriend or husband/wife.

Relationships can be very hard for people with Asperger Syndrome. They are often easy in the beginning, as we are able to put on a façade of sorts and to really just enjoy the moment and be social and interact with the person we are dating. Unfortunately, as relationships turn serious and we begin to spend more time together, the ability to put on an act or to work incredibly hard at saying and doing the right thing 24/7 becomes overwhelming and impossible.

One thing to note is that while a relationship in its infancy may be easy, finding a relationship is often difficult for females with AS. Our awkwardness and our tendency to dress more for comfort than fashion and to not overly worry about appearance can make it harder for us to be noticed by potential partners. With that said, however, many Aspies can and do find partners that they love and who love them in return.

There are some concerns that come with relationships for women on the autism spectrum. One of the biggest is that our awkwardness and our personalities often attract those who are abusive and who can sense that we can be easily manipulated. This is especially true in first relationships, when many Aspies feel happy just to have someone and do not know that there are others out there who will love us for who we are. Domestic and sexual violence against female Aspies is common, and it is something that you should never, ever put up with. Change may be hard, especially when you love someone, but getting out of a situation like that is essential for both your safety and your physical and emotional health.

Another concern for many women on the spectrum is becoming obsessive. We tend to throw ourselves wholeheartedly into anything that interests us. While this might be wonderful when we are talking about a hobby like playing the piano, it can be bothersome and even stalker-like when it comes to relationships. Calling multiple times a day, checking up on a partner, or spending so much time with them that they are unable to engage with their own friends can be detrimental to the relationship, even if it feels wonderful to the AS partner. Allowing your NT partner the chance to get out and socialize is important, especially because the chances are good that they will end up playing both the role of best friend and significant other in your life. Living with an Aspie can be hard, and our partners need someone outside of the relationship to talk to when things get tough.

Aspie or NT?

One question that many of us ask is whether it would be better to date another Aspie or someone who is neurotypical. The answer is really that both can have their advantages and disadvantages and that what you should be looking for is someone who loves and respects you as you are.

Dating another Aspie can be wonderful in that you understand one another's needs and limitations. You both speak honestly and bluntly. You can click on a level that is very difficult with an NT partner. It can also prove stressful, however, when you have different routine needs, special interests, and focal points. Like with any other relationship, an Aspie to Aspie relationship is a matter of finding out whether or not the two of you are a good fit together, despite how much it seems you already have in common.

Dating a neurotypical can also have many advantages, especially if you find someone who is willing to become educated about Asperger Syndrome. As Aspies, there are simply certain areas of life, such as social navigation, where we have difficulties and deficits. By choosing an NT partner, you are potentially choosing someone who has strength in areas that are weak for you, just as your AS gifts may give you strengths in areas where your partner is weak such as problem solving, technical work, or some other area of passion and interest.

For me, my relationships have all been with NT partners. This hasn't been a choice, however, as I really never knew about AS and certainly didn't know until I was already married that I had it. The diagnosis has certainly helped me see where and why other relationships went wrong, and it has helped me to be a better wife to my partner. I think our differences make us stronger as a couple. While it might seem nice to think of someone who cherishes routine and other things the way I do, I can't imagine a more loving relationship and truly feel that nobody could ever understand me the way that my wife does.

Advice

If you are considering entering into a relationship, there is much advice to be sought. For starters, it is important to find someone who is interested in you as you are and who is not looking to change you. You deserve someone who is willing to learn more about Asperger Syndrome and who will work to navigate life with your needs in mind.

For those dating an NT partner, it is also important to remember that your partner does not have AS. This means that he or she may not have the same need for routine or the same aversion to change as you. It also means that he or she may not share your passions when it comes to special interests. While it is certainly important to have big things in common, it is equally important to remember to afford your partner the independence they need in order to thrive, even when this is difficult or seems to interfere with the way you want your relationship to work.

There is much advice that can be offered to women seeking to enter into relationships, and one thing it is important to be clear with your partner about is your needs. This includes more than just your needs for routine and planning, but your needs for control in some areas of life, your need for honesty at all costs, and other uniquely Aspie needs.

It is also important to remember that relationships are two-sided. This means that as much as you will need your partner to work to understand you, you are going to have to work to understand your partner. Relationships are never smooth sailing 100% of the time, but learning how to meet your partner's needs is crucial. For example, while many Aspie women are happy with only their partner for social interaction, most NT partners will want and need to maintain many friendships in their lives. This is an important thing for them, and we must learn to accommodate it.

We must also learn how to communicate with our partners and show affection in clear ways. It doesn't always occur to women on the spectrum to say I love you or to offer hugs and kisses for no reason, yet these acts play a large role in relationships. Showing affection and letting our partners know how we feel is critical, just as it is critical to let them know when something is bothering us. It is easy to expect our partners to pick up on signs when something is wrong, but this is really more like baiting a trap and it is likely to end in a meltdown. Just as we can't always read our partners, they can't always read us, either.

While I have already touched on this, the single biggest piece of advice that I can offer is to be safe. There are many people out there who prey on people with AS and other autism spectrum disorders because we can be easily manipulated. Violence and abuse, including verbal abuse, are never okay and should never be tolerated in any relationship.

Parenting

Parenting can be a big struggle for anyone, and it can be especially hard on those with AS. In fact, many NT partners end up feeling as though they do a majority of the parenting in a household where one partner has AS and the other does not. With that said, however, parenting can be a source of great joy for those with AS.

One thing that I hear frequently from people with AS is that they simply do not feel a bond with their children as infants. While this may sound horrifying to many NT parents, for those of us on the spectrum, we want someone with whom we can interact. A baby, in many ways, is a small being that simply cries, eats, sleeps, poops, and remains a complete mystery. They can be a source of anxiety and fear, even when we love them unconditionally. If you are a new parent feeling these sorts of emotions, it is important to realize that these feelings will change as your child starts to communicate and show personality.

My experiences as a parent are somewhat limited, as my kids were 8 and 10 when they came into my life. Yet I can say that it took time to create a parental bond. It was very hard for me to learn not to see the kids as little friends and to take on the role of mother- something that is very hard for many on the spectrum.

Parenting difficulties are not at all uncommon for those of us on the spectrum, and they come in many forms. For some, there is an inherent inability to handle the sound of crying or yelling without becoming overstimulated, while for others, helping with homework that seems so crystal clear can be a major source of anxiety and stress. Aspies are by nature very self-focused, and having a being entirely dependent on you can be an anxiety provoking experience that takes a lot of help to overcome.

While this may sound negative, there is nothing quite like being a parent. Children can give your life a brand new meaning and can motivate you to better deal with AS and all of the things that come along with it. Special interests are things that you can share with your own kids, helping build things in common and helping to enhance the bonding experience. For example, my kids are near-experts at sanding, staining, and refinishing furniture, and Monkey Boy has memorized virtually all of the rules of NFL football just by watching games with me. Remember that AS bestows upon you many unique traits and gifts that, if aimed in the right direction, can make you in some ways a more unique and exciting parent than many who are not on the spectrum.

Advice

There are many people who are on the spectrum who do not desire children, and it is important to realize that we no longer live in a society where childless or even unwed women are frowned upon socially. For those who do want children, however, it is important to understand what a lifelong commitment a child truly is. A child is not just someone you raise until they are 18, they are someone that you will love and for whom you will provide care for the rest of your life. You won't just be there for diaper changes, first days of school, big dances, and graduation. You will also be expected to be there for college, breakups, marriage, and many other life events as well as holidays.

Other advice I can offer comes from personal experience. In a previous chapter, I recommended creating a sensory space within your home. I feel that this is especially necessary if you have children. Not only does it afford you a place of respite if things with your kids become overwhelming (assuming you have a partner who can assume the parental role while you de-stress or that your children are old enough to be left alone briefly), but it gives you a place to safely retreat when you are on the verge of a tantrum or a meltdown. Children see and hear more than we realize sometimes, and while we want to educate them as much as possible about AS, it is critical that we do what we can to shield them from the chaos and destruction (either verbal or physical) of a meltdown.

For those of you with a partner to help in parenting, it can help to assign duties. If you enjoy helping with homework, taking care of your child's bedtime routine, or some other aspects of care, make a pledge to be responsible for these things while asking your partner to help with things that you are unable to handle. An NT partner should never feel like a single parent with you in the house, and it is equally important that your kids never feel as though they have only one parent when there are two of you to show love and to share in special moments.

Speaking of special moments, self-focus can be a big problem for some AS moms, especially those with NT children. While many parents see inherently the importance of getting a child ready for picture day, attending yet another Little League practice, or taking photos before a big dance, many of us simply do not think of these things as life-altering events. Remember that there are many moments that are special to your child and make sure that you are a part of the memories that they are building as often as possible. It helps to strengthen the parent-child bond and can often help resolve feelings of detachment that are common among parents who have AS as well as their children.

Another area where self-focus can impact parenting is in the area of a child's social development. Having sleepovers, taking your child to basketball practice every day, or ensuring that your child has an active social and extracurricular life is important, even when it is difficult. It can be hard for many Aspie moms to remember that their children have deep social needs, but it is a critical thing to actively work on.

As a last piece of advice for those of you considering becoming a mother, it is important to understand the risk of passing down AS or autism to your child. While this may be seen as a blessing to some, it can come as a total shock to others. There is a strong genetic link when it comes to autism spectrum disorders, and being prepared to raise a child on the spectrum can save you a lot of stress and even help you know to look for warning signs as your child starts to grow up. By looking for early warning signs, you can provide your child with the early diagnosis that many of us never had, ensuring that they have supports in place from an early age and ensuring that you as a parent have extra supports as well.

Employment

Finding and maintaining a job can be hard for many women with AS. While we have an easier time fitting in socially, we still have a hard time with prolonged socialization, interacting with strangers, and of course, sensory stimuli.

For many Aspies, myself included, the choice is to become a freelancer or start a business. When you are your own boss and get to call the shots, you can manage your triggers, find a job that suits your special skills and interests, and take time off when you are feeling overwhelmed without the risk of being fired. Freelancing work can come in many forms, from writing to technical support, computer work, web design, handywoman services, and much more.

For other women with AS, however, starting a business is either undesirable or not an option. It is important to know that in most cases, you **can** work and maintain a job- it is all in the job that you choose.

One piece of advice that I recommend is finding a job that matches your skills and interests. If you despise talking on the phone, a job that makes this a main part of your duties is likely to cause a great deal of anxiety and stress for you. Take the time to consider the attributes you are looking for in a job as well as your own strengths and deficits and try to find a career path that will lead to sustainable and enjoyable employment.

Another thing that you can do is to make your boss and coworkers aware of your condition if you think that it will be well received. While they may not be able to do much about the hum of fluorescent lights or the smells that come from the break room, they may be able to accommodate an inability to multitask and even to use it to their advantage. It may be uncomfortable to let those in your workplace know that you have AS, and it is always your decision, but in the right workplace, it can create a better environment for you, your employer, and your co-workers.

Depression and Anxiety

Depression and anxiety are two conditions that can occur frequently in women with Asperger Syndrome. In fact, they are so common that they are practically symptoms of the disorder. One reason for this is that we simply aren't wired to handle changes and setbacks as readily as our neurotypical peers, although genes, brain chemistry, life history, and many other factors often come into play.

Depression in someone with AS can be serious, and it can be triggered by many things. Ridicule by peers, money or legal problems, a difficult relationship, or even a meltdown can be enough to trigger the spiral into depression. Knowing when you are starting to feel depressed and taking action to stop it can be critical in ending the cycle.

If you are just starting to experience depression, you can try things such as exercising, eating healthier, and talking to a supportive friend, family member, or therapist. All of these things are shown to help alleviate depression in different ways. In fact, exercise and a healthy diet can also help prevent depression, as can a healthy social life and a therapist trained in either talk therapy or CBT.

If your depression has slipped out of control and you are not eating, not getting out of bed or not sleeping, or have thoughts of suicide, it may be important to take more drastic and urgent steps. Calling your therapist for extra sessions is certainly recommended, and speaking with your psychiatrist if you are on medication for depression is essential.

NOTE If you are experiencing thoughts of suicide, even if you do not believe you will act on them, **please** call your local crisis line, contact your therapist after hours, or seek help at your local emergency room.

Signs of Depression

- Not eating or eating too much
- Rapid weight gain or loss
- Loss of interest in pleasurable activities
- Loss of interest in friends and loved ones
- Sleeping too much or not enough
- Suicidal thoughts and ideations

Anxiety is another hallmark symptom for many women with Asperger Syndrome. It can present in a myriad of ways, from physical symptoms and illness to changes in your mental state, fears and phobias, and more. CBT can be an excellent way to handle anxiety, and yoga and mindfulness practice have shown great benefit in reducing overall levels of anxiety. Like with depression, exercise, diet, socialization, and therapy can all help alleviate symptoms.

Symptoms of Anxiety

What follows are some of the most common symptoms of anxiety

- Racing or pounding heartbeat
- Sweating
- Physical illness or somatic symptoms
- Nervousness
- Panic
- A sensation of being unable to catch your breath
- Chest pain

For women with Asperger's Syndrome, anxiety can also manifest in other ways. Many people who are experiencing intense anxiety may become much more rigid and controlling in their routines and may be much more vulnerable to meltdowns when these routines are broken. They may melt down more easily and more intensely and may become more preoccupied with their special interest. These are important symptoms to note and to speak about with your therapist, and they can be crucial symptoms to share with your partner or roommates.

Advice

Dealing with anxiety and depression in the short term can be accomplished at home. Getting through a tough moment can be done using CBT, exercising, or even by spending time in the company of loved ones or friends. If you are experiencing anxiety and/or depression, however, it is crucial that you take the time to speak with your therapist. These conditions are very common in people with AS and they can be treated either via therapy or, less commonly, with medication. Whatever you do, don't remain silent. Too many Aspies commit suicide every year due to depression and anxiety symptoms that can be treated with the right help.

Bullying and Abuse

When most people think of bullying and abuse, they think of children. While children are in fact commonly bullied and abused, especially children with special needs, it is all too common for women on the spectrum to find themselves victims of abuse as well. Bullying in the workplace, among peers, and in relationships is all too common. Our quirks and differences make us easy targets, and in relationships they make it easy for partners to see that we will often put up with abusive behavior rather than to experience the change that comes with leaving the relationship.

There are many different types of abuse that are common among women on the spectrum. As mentioned, workplace and peer bullying and verbal abuse are very common. It is also important to note that women on the spectrum are more susceptible to sexual abuse, both at the hands of partners as well as strangers and even sometimes friends or family members.

It is easy to say that no type of bullying or abuse should ever be endured, but it is a much harder thing indeed to act on that thought. Leaving a job or a relationship means making a major change, and many relationships involve giving up someone you love and possibly even fighting for custody of your children. It can be easy to worry that AS will mean that you will lose a battle against an abusive partner, but it is never a reason to stay in the relationship. If children are involved, it is crucial that you get them out of the abusive home as quickly as possible, even if they are not themselves the victims of abuse.

With my first girlfriend, our relationship was very volatile and abusive. There were countless times that we would get into fights, even after her son was born and living with us. It took us years to realize that we simply could not live together and we both carry many mental and emotional scars as a result of our time together. While we separated when he was still very small, I worry to this day about the effect that it had on him.

On a different note, there are many people with Asperger Syndrome who are bullies or abusers themselves. Meltdowns are a common part of AS and are to be expected, but many women with AS, especially those with anxiety, are prone to exploding at loved ones and saying or doing harmful things. If you find that you are bullying your loved ones, it is important to seek help. When I first met my wife, my meltdowns were almost always aimed in her direction and I would say terrible, terrible things to her. When we would disagree and the tension would escalate, I would eventually resort to name-calling and other bullying behaviors. It took a great deal of hard work and therapy to understand that I was taking things out on her because I saw her as a safe place and a great deal more work to learn to take my meltdowns to a separate and private room rather than yelling.

Advice

If you are the victim of abuse or bullying, it is your job and your duty to report it. While this may seem intimidating or even dangerous, it can be the only way to protect yourself. If you are being harassed in the workplace, inform your supervisor of what is going on and make it clear that you will not remain with the company if the perpetrator is allowed to remain.

If you are in a relationship, talking to your therapist can be crucial when verbal abuse is present. If you are being physically or sexually abused, contact your local battered women's shelter or contact the police, who will be able to help you find a safe place to stay until you are able to find a place of your own. Staying in an abusive relationship may seem like the best thing for the kids or the most stable thing for you, but it is truly dangerous and can lead to escalation as well as the development of PTSD for both you and any children present.

Getting the Right Help

Whether you are diagnosed with Asperger Syndrome or simply strongly suspect that you have it, finding the right help is crucial in building the skills you need in order to better overcome the differences that can set you apart from the NT world. While the AS community is a proud one and we like to celebrate our unique qualities, finding someone to help with problems in relationships, at work, and in other areas of life can be crucial.

There is a great deal of debate over the importance of diagnosis in adults. The diagnosis of AS can be very costly and difficult to obtain, and many adults have found ways of fitting in that mask many of the criteria used to diagnose the condition. Whether or not you decide to seek a formal diagnosis is up to you, but finding a care provider, whether psychiatrist, psychologist, or therapist who understands your unique differences and challenges is crucial.

The wrong provider and the wrong diagnosis can sometimes do more harm than good. I have had a psychiatrist who did little more than tell me stories about all of her other patients. I have been given many wrong diagnoses that led to medications that nearly killed me or caused me to kill myself. I have even had a therapist who assured me that my aversion to strong smells, especially in the kitchen, was a clear sign that I had a trauma in my kitchen as a child that I just couldn't remember. Yet for all of these bad experiences, finding the right provider can make all the difference in the world.

When seeking a provider, it is important to consider your unique needs. If you are looking to go back to work, someone with an understanding of AS who works in vocational rehabilitation might be the perfect fit for you, while someone struggling with meltdowns or depression might work better with a therapist who specializes in CBT.

For many Aspies, a psychiatrist is also highly recommended. Not only are there medications available that can lessen the severity and duration of meltdowns, but AS is often comorbid with other disorders. ADHD, depression, anxiety, bipolar disorder, PTSD, and many other conditions are often found in women who are diagnosed with Asperger Syndrome.

If you already have a therapist or psychiatrist who works with you and who is a good fit for you, a diagnosis is no reason to switch to a specialist. If, however, you find that your current provider is not a good fit or you simply do not have one, calling around or looking online for a database of adult Asperger specialists can be a very valuable tool, especially one who has worked with women on the spectrum. It can be very hard to find someone who works especially with people on the spectrum, or even who has experience working with Aspies, but it is well worth the hard work and effort, even if it takes months of calling and reaching dead ends.

The Gifts of Asperger Syndrome

While much of this book has been a survival guide for women with Asperger's Syndrome, it is important that we take time to celebrate the gifts that AS brings to us.

It has been my belief since I first learned about AS that being wired differently is indeed a gift. I have always felt emotions more strongly and more intensely than those around me, even though I rarely have the means of expressing them. In times of joy and great accomplishment, and even in times where I simply feel satisfied, this is truly a blessing.

I also think that all women with Asperger Syndrome are blessed with gifts that are unique to themselves. Maybe you can write amazing novels or maybe you can play the piano like a virtuoso. Maybe you are excellent at doing things that make others happy, or maybe you have some other gift. Whatever your talent or gift may be, rest assured that it is there, even if you have yet to find it. I didn't discover writing as a career until I was in my 30's!

Asperger Syndrome brings us many challenges in our daily lives, but it gives us an insight and rational way of looking at the world that most people don't get to experience. It is important that we always remember this, especially in the hard times, as AS gives us something that nobody outside the spectrum will ever experience.

Conclusion

It is my deepest hope that this book has provided you with a greater understanding of AS and how to handle it. I also hope that you have enjoyed reading my story and learning about my life. This book is intended as the start of a series of survival guides, and I hope that you have enjoyed it enough that you will want to continue reading the series as it progresses. For those of you who feel that I have not gone into enough detail on certain aspects of AS, take heart, as many of the topics broached in this book will be made into their own full books in the months and years to come.

Glossary of Terms

Here, I want to present a glossary of terms used throughout this book, as well as other terms often associated with Asperger's Syndrome.

Alexithymia or Emotion Blindness- difficulty or an inability to identify and describe emotions

Asperger Syndrome or Asperger's Syndrome- a disorder on the autism spectrum that creates notable social difficulties.

Aspie- a term often used to denote someone with Asperger's Syndrome

CBT- Cognitive Behavior Therapy, or a therapy that works to change behaviors by identifying and changing the thoughts that precede them. This technique is shown to be highly helpful in alleviating distress and addressing both behavior and social issues.

DSM- the Diagnostic and Statistical Manual of Mental Disorders, a guidebook for diagnosing autism spectrum disorders, anxiety, depression, and other neurological and mental health disorders

Empathy- the ability to understand the emotions of others and respond appropriately. Displays of empathy are often difficult, if not impossible, for those on the spectrum, even when deep feelings are present.

Face Blindness-an inability to recognize faces, even familiar ones. This is a common trait among people on the spectrum, although not a universal one.

Meltdown- a situation where the Aspie temporarily loses control of her emotions and actions. This is typically due to a number of stressors that can be emotional or sensory in nature. A meltdown often looks to others like a tantrum and may involve the Aspie crying, engaging in self-harming behaviors, yelling, or even fully retreating and shutting down.

Mind Blindness- the inability to read facial cues and to pick up on social cues or on the nuances of verbal and facial expressions of others

Neurotypical, or NT- a person with typical neurological and social development, someone most people would define as "normal".

Ritual or Routine- a set of behaviors performed in order to avoid anxiety and distress. Some examples include a daily regimen or plan, bedtime routines, repetitive activities, the need to repeat a set of specific movements or noises, or any other routine that is needed to help alleviate or prevent distress.

Self Harming Behavior- behavior such as head banging or biting that is harmful to the Aspie. This often occurs during a meltdown and can be among the most difficult symptoms to control.

Sensory Stimuli- any stimuli that affects one of the five main senses, such as a scent, a bright light or bright colors, noises, etc.

Sensory Overload- when the Aspie has had too much sensory input to process. This can easily lead to a meltdown or shutdown and should be avoided when possible.

Sensory Kit- a kit that includes tools to help prevent sensory overload. Tools may include earplugs, a face mask, tactile objects or any other tools that the Aspie finds helpful.

Stim- a repetitive behavior that is self-stimulating, such as tapping, rocking, head banging, spinning, or humming. This can help Aspies to regulate their emotions and to deal with stress.

Theory of Mind- the ability to attribute a mental state or emotion to oneself and to then understand that others may have a different belief or mental state and attempt to predict their behavior. This ability is often lacking in people on the autism spectrum.

Resources

www.help4aspergrs.com- a website run by renowned Aspie author Rudy Simone

Tony Attwood- *The Complete Guide to Asperger Syndrome* 2006

Nick Dubin- *Asperger Syndrome and Anxiety: A Guide to Successful Stress Management* 2009 www.wrongplanet.net- a forum for people with ASDs as well as for professionals and parents who work with these individuals

Valerie L. Gaus, PhD- *Living Well on the Spectrum* 2011

Rudy Simone- *22 Things a Woman With Asperger's Syndrome Wants Her Partner to Know* 2012

Acknowledgements

I wish to thank everyone who has helped me in the writing of this book. To my faithful wife, who not only endures me, but loves me and even helped me edit and revise this book, I thank you. My two beautiful children, Monkey Boy and The Girl, you are my entire world, even if I never let you read this book. To my many, many Kickstarter backers- you made this possible. I can't believe how many of you there were or how generous you were, even those of you I don't know. Thank you. To my mother, my brother, my Grandpa, Mrs. Betty, and Gramma and Papa, thank you for loving me both because of and often in spite of my differences, my meltdowns, and my quirks. And to all of you who purchase and read these pages, thank you. I sincerely hope that you have enjoyed them.

Printed in Great Britain
by Amazon